I0701474

INTRODUCTION

Saxenda (liraglutide) is a prescription medicine permitted through the Food and Drug Administration (FDA) as part of a broader weight loss plan that includes a healthful weight-reduction plan and regular bodily pastime. It belongs to a class of medicine known as GLP-1 receptor agonists. These pills mimic glucagon-like peptide 1, a hormone that regulates urge for food, ensuing in decreased hunger and decreased calorie consumption. Saxenda is available in prefilled multidose injection pens to deliver an everyday subcutaneous injection for your belly, thigh, or upper arm. The starting dose is zero.6 milligrams (mg), which you may boom to 3 mg for protection.

WHO CAN USE IT?

Doctors may additionally prescribe Saxenda for adults with a frame mass index (BMI) of 30 kilograms consistent with square meter (kg/m2) or higher, or 27 kg/m2 or better and as a minimum one weight-related situation, including high blood strain, type 2 diabetes, or high ldl cholesterol. It's also accepted for children ages 12–17 with a body weight above 132 pounds (lb) [60 kilograms (kg)] and a BMI of 30 kg/m2, to help them shed pounds and maintain their weight.

But it's not pretty much numbers on a scale. Saxenda is supposed for those with issue dropping weight thru food regimen and exercise by me and who can also want extra aid to efficaciously control their weight. If you're considering Saxenda, it's important to discuss it with your healthcare professional to fully apprehend the blessings and any potential risks and to make sure it aligns with your health profile and weight control desires.

SAXENDA SIDE OUTCOMES

While Saxenda may be a powerful tool for weight control, it does have some capacity aspect results, together with:

- Nausea and vomiting

- Stomach pain

- Constipation or diarrhea

- Heartburn, indigestion, or GERD

- bloating and belching

- Headache

- Fatigue

- Dizziness

- temper adjustments

- Drug interactions

- Redness, swelling, and pain at the injection web site

- Low blood sugar

Some much less commonplace but more extreme facet results may include:

- Hypersensitive reaction (anaphylaxis)

- Pancreatitis

- Gallstones (acute cholelithiasis)

- Acute kidney injury and kidney failure

- Modifications in heart fee

- Suicidal conduct or ideation

- Risk of thyroid C-cellular tumors When the use of Saxenda, hold a near eye on your fitness. Report any concerning signs and symptoms on your healthcare professional without delay. They can provide extra special statistics and assist manage any side consequences, ensuring your remedy plan is secure and powerful.

HOW TO GET SAXENDA

You can go to a healthcare professional in individual or use a telehealth platform to gain a prescription for Saxenda. In man or woman Meeting with a healthcare professional to get a Saxenda prescription has several advantages over telehealth alternatives. You'll advantage from a comprehensive bodily examination, including blood pressure and other crucial signal readings, and the possibility to ask questions and discuss alternatives.

Your healthcare expert also can order lab paintings to evaluate your blood and metabolic markers to determine if Saxenda is suitable. They can then tailor a diet regime specifically to your needs. Furthermore, in-person visits allow for more effective follow-up and closer development tracking. You'll also have access to supplementary resources like nutrition and workout steering. Start the manner with the aid of deciding on a healthcare expert with know-how in weight management. Your number one care company can offer a referral in case you're uncertain where to start. Should you and your healthcare expert agree that Saxenda is appropriate, you'll get a

prescription to fill at the pharmacy
of your desire.

ARE WEIGHT LOSS MEDICATIONS EFFECTIVE? A DIETITIAN EXPLAINS

Prescription weight loss medicines, consisting of GLP-1 agonists, orlistat, and setmelanotide, may be effective for some human beings. But other lifestyle adjustments are still vital for long-time period success. If it's hard to shed pounds notwithstanding making adjustments for your food regimen and growing your bodily activity, you'll be questioning whether a prescription weight loss medication is right for you.

These medicines have a tendency to work through one or more of those mechanisms:

• reducing urge for food, making you feels fuller, so that you devour less energy

• reducing the absorption of vitamins, which include fat, making you is taking in fewer calories

• Growing metabolism, making you burn more energy

When paired with other life-style changes and brought beneath the supervision of a healthcare professional, these tablets may provide an effective manner to decrease your weight. We reviewed all the weight loss medicinal drugs that are currently available, along with how they paintings, who they is probably suitable for, studies on their effectiveness, and capability safety concerns.

WHAT MEDICATIONS ARE FDA APPROVED FOR WEIGHT REDUCTION?

The Food and Drug Administration (FDA) has approved several pills for dropping weight with obese and obesity. These medicines require a prescription from a medical doctor and have to only be taken beneath clinical supervision. These currently includeTrusted Source:

- GLP-1 agonists, which includes liraglutide (Saxenda), semaglutide (Wegovy), and tirzepatide (Zepbound)

- orlistat (Xenical)

- phentermine/topiramate (Qsymia)

- naltrexone/bupropion (Contrave)

- setmelanotide (Imcivree)

- Appetite suppressants, inclusive of phentermine (Adipex-P or Lomaira)

These medicines should be combined with a balanced weight loss food regimen, as by me, they're not probable a useful long-time period answer for weight problems and might cause weight regain through the years.

They also have many viable aspect consequences, some of which may be extreme.

HOW EFFECTIVE ARE PRESCRIPTION WEIGHT LOSS CAPSULES?

Weight loss medicinal drugs may be a powerful device to assist weight management. Most paintings by decreasing your food consumption, reducing fat absorption, or growing metabolism, ensuing in giant weight loss over time.

In most cases, those prescription medications can generally bring about around five–10percentTrusted Source weight loss. However, this could range depending on several elements, along with the unique remedy which you take. Keep in mind that these medications should be used along nutritional adjustments and life-style adjustments, which includes ordinary physical interest. Not only will adopting nutritional and way of life changes help increase the effectiveness of weight loss tablets, however they'll also help minimize weight regain, which frequently occurs when you forestall taking these medicinal drugs.

GLP-1 AGONISTS

Three GLP-1 agonists were authorized for weight loss, along with liraglutide (Saxenda), semaglutide (Wegovy), and tirzepatide (Zepbound). All 3 are available as a self-administered injection, but liraglutide is administered once daily, while semaglutide and tirzepatide are best injected once consistent with week. Though now not permitted specifically for weight reduction, a few different GLP-1 agonists intended to deal with kind 2 diabetes are now and again prescribed off-label for weight control, includingTrusted Source:

- semaglutide (Ozempic or Rybelsus)

- dulaglutide (Trulicity)

- liraglutide (Victoza)

- exenatide (Byetta)

- exenatide extended-launch (Bydureon BCise)

- tirzepatide (Mounjaro)

GLP-1 agonists are simplest available through a prescription from a health practitioner or other certified healthcare professional. Several telehealth offerings and weight loss packages may also provide prescriptions in case you meet the eligibility criteria. How it works: GLP-1 agonists paintings by means of slowingTrusted Source the emptying of the stomach, increasing feelings of fullness, and decreasing the secretion of glucagon, a hormone involved in regulating urge for food. Effectiveness: Several researches have discovered that GLP-1 agonists can be useful for weight control. For example, one examine with 1,961 adults determined that taking 2.4 milligrams (mg) of semaglutide per week mixed with way of life changes resulted in a nearly 15p.CTrusted Source reduction in body weight after 68 weeks. Another small take a look at found that human beings taking liraglutide lost an average of 17.2 lb (7.8 kg) Trusted Source over 6 months. More lately, a 2023 segment three clinical trial in 2,539 adults located that people taking tirzepatide lost 20% or greater in their weight over the path of seventy two weeks. Side consequences: Common facet results includeTrusted Source nausea, vomiting, diarrhea, dizziness, headaches, elevated coronary heart fee, infections, and indigestion.

Though uncommon, severe aspect effects have additionally been reported, which may require clinical interest? These include kidney problems, thyroid C-cell tumors, gallbladder disease, low blood sugar, and suicidal ideation. It's critical to be in regular contact along with your healthcare professional to monitor for those aspect results. More studies is likewise needed at the long-time period effects of those medications, as there's problem approximately capacity weight regain through the years.

Contraindications: This medication isn't always

recommendedTrusted Source for human beings with more than one endocrine neoplasia (MEN) syndrome kind 2, records of thyroid most cancers or pancreatitis, being pregnant, and current use of positive prescription medicines. Additionally, people with intense gastrointestinal conditionsTrusted Source, inclusive of gastroparesis and inflammatory bowel disorder must keep away from taking GLP-1 agonists. Jargon-buster: "Contraindications" are any reason that someone shouldn't take a particular medicine.

ORLISTAT (XENICAL)

Orlistat is an oral medication that's available through prescription as Xenical. It also can be purchased over the counter as the brand Alli. After a medical session, a medical doctor can prescribe orlistat. Certain telehealth services can also offer a prescription for this medication.

How it really works: Orlistat works through blocking the interest of certain enzymes used to break down fats in the digestive tract, which helps to reduceTrusted Source the quantity of calories you take in.

Effectiveness: According to a 2011 studyTrusted Source of eighty human beings with weight problems, folks who took orlistat lost an average of 10.Three kilos (lb), or four.Sixty five kilograms (kg), after 6 months. They additionally experienced large discounts in frame mass index (BMI), belly fat, and total and LDL (bad) cholesterol levels. Side effects: Orlistat frequently reasons digestive issues like free or oily stools, gasoline, and frequent bowel actions, making the medication difficult for some people to tolerate. It could also make a contribution to nutrient deficiencies, which include in fat-soluble nutrients A, D, E, or K.

Following a low fat eating regimen is typically encouraged at the same time as taking this remedy to assist decrease destructive side consequences. Contraindications: continual malabsorption, cholestasis (a type of liver sickness), pregnancy, renal impairment, and contemporary use of certain prescription medicinal drugs.

PHENTERMINE/TOPIRAMATE (QSYMIA)

Phentermine/topiramate is an oral medicine that requires a prescription from a physician and is sold below the logo Qsymia.How it works: This remedy includesTrusted Source phentermine, an important apprehensive device stimulant and appetite suppressant with comparable mechanisms to amphetamine. It additionally consists of topiramate, an anticonvulsant that helps reduce appetite and beautify satiety (feeling full) to sell weight reduction.

Effectiveness: One studies overview concluded that phentermine/topiramate ended in an average weight loss of 17 lb (7.7 kg) Trusted Source and substantially decreased stomach fats, blood strain, blood sugar, and levels of cholesterol. Another assessment evaluating the effectiveness of several weight loss medications found that humans with obese or obesity who took phentermine/topiramate lost a mean of 19.Four lb (eight.Eight kg) Trusted Source after 1 12 months.

Side effects: The maximum commonTrusted Source facet consequences related to phentermine/topiramate encompass dry mouth, constipation, and a sensation of pins and needles (paresthesia). It can also cause increased body temperature, and lack of ability to sweat, and psychiatric or cognitive disturbances. Contraindications: This medicinal drug isn't advocated for people with glaucoma (eye situations that can lead to blindness), records of hyperthyroidism, being pregnant, latest use of monoamine oxidase inhibitors, and present day use of certain prescription medications.

NALTREXONE/BUPROPION (CONTRAVE)

This medication, offered beneath the name Contrave, is an oral medicinal drug that combinesTrusted Source bupropion, an antidepressant, and naltrexone, which is used to manage opioid or alcohol use disease. A doctor can determine whether or not Contrave may be a great choice for you after which offer a prescription. Some on-line services may additionally prescribe Contrave following a digital session with a healthcare professional.

How it really works: Though the exact mechanism of naltrexone/bupropion isn't completely understood, it's believed to promoteTrusted Source weight loss via performing on sure components of the mind to lessen meals consumption, increase metabolism, and growth feelings of fullness. Effectiveness: One evaluate of 4 studies showed that naltrexone/bupropion was related to vast weight loss compared with a placebo, with participants losing a median of eleven–22 lb (5–9 kg)Trusted Source.

Another review had similar findings, reporting that naltrexone/bupropion can be effectiveTrusted Source for long-time period weight reduction preservation as properly. Side outcomes: Naltrexone/bupropion may additionally causeTrusted Source nausea, constipation, headache, vomiting, dizziness, dry mouth, diarrhea, and insomnia. It may also growth coronary heart charge and blood pressure. Contraindications: This medicinal drug isn't always advocated for humans with records of seizures, give up-stage renal sickness, pregnancy, and cutting-edge use of monoamine oxidase inhibitors, opioids, or positive different prescription medications.

SETMELANOTIDE (IMCIVREE)

Setmelanotide, bought as Imcivree, is in a class of medications referred to as melanocortin 4 (MC4) receptor agonists. It's an injectable medication approvedTrusted Source for treating obesity caused by positive genetic mutations and is to be had most effective through prescription. How it works: People with precise genetic mutations may additionally revel in insufficient activation of melanocortin receptorsTrusted Source in the mind that may contribute to weight problems.

Setmelanotide works by way of increasing the activation of these receptors, leading to decreased starvation, reduced calorie intake, and accelerated metabolism, all of which could promote weight reduction. Effectiveness: One take a look at in 21 people taking setmelanotide observed that round 62percentTrusted Source of contributors executed as a minimum 10% weight reduction after 1 year. Participants additionally experienced a huge discount in starvation with no critical treatment-associated unfavorable events suggested.

Another small have a look at in kids, adolescents, and adults foundTrusted Source that setmelanotide considerably progressed first-rate of life as early as 5 weeks after beginning remedy, which will be associated with decreased hunger and frame weight. Side results: Some of the maximum common aspect consequences of setmelanotide consist of injection website reactions, hyperpigmentation, nausea, headache, diarrhea, and belly or returned ache. Fatigue, vomiting, and melancholy have also been reported.

Contraindications: This remedy isn't always endorsed for humans with renal impairment, and people who are pregnant or breastfeeding.

WHO ARE WEIGHT LOSS TABLETS FOR?

Most weight reduction medications are approvedTrusted Source for adults with weight problems or with overweight and at the least one weight-associated condition, which includes:

- Kind 2 diabetes

- Excessive blood strain

- High ldl cholesterol

Similarly, setmelanotide (Imcivree) is intendedTrusted Source to deal with obesity caused by certain genetic issues.

These medicines are designed for those who haven't been able to acquire weight reduction via other strategies, including diet or life-style adjustments. Though they shouldn't be considered a short restoration, those medicinal drugs may be a useful device to help weight management when mixed with normal physical hobby and a nutritious food plan. Keep in thoughts that weight reduction medications aren't appropriate for every person, such as people who are pregnant, those with certain health situations, or people taking precise medicinal drugs.

A healthcare professional can offer steering on whether you is probably a candidate for a prescription, relying on your non-public desires, scientific history, and health reputation.

THE BOTTOM LINE
Prescription medicinal drugs have robust proof to guide their effectiveness for meaningful weight reduction. However, it's essential to bear in mind eligibility criteria, ability aspect outcomes, and whether or not they're indicated for lengthy-time period use. Additionally, though they can promote weight loss and can even offer other health advantages, observe that these medications are not suitable for absolutely everyone and might result in weight regain once you forestall taking them.

A physician or different relied on healthcare expert let you decide that's proper for you and the way to include it into a healthy weight management plan. Finally, it's vital to bear in mind that those products should no longer be considered a "short restoration" for weight reduction. Obesity is a continual condition, and medicinal drugs can be just one a part of a remedy plan to help acquire and preserve weight reduction. Instead, they have to be used best as directed and paired with a balanced weight loss program, wholesome life-style, and normal physical interest for quality results.

THE END

www.ingramcontent.com/pod-product-compliance
Lightning Source LLC
Chambersburg PA
CBHW051923250726

48659CB00002B/816